MEDITATION FOR BEGINNERS

a. Habib

Chapter 1: about meditation

Meditation is an approach to training the mind, similar to the way that fitness is an approach to training the body. But many meditation techniques exist — so how do you learn how to meditate?

"In Buddhist tradition, the word 'meditation' is equivalent to a word like 'sports' in the U.S. It's a family of activities, not a single thing," University of Wisconsin neuroscience lab director Richard J. Davidson, Ph.D., told The New York Times. And different meditation practices require different mental skills.

It's extremely difficult for a beginner to sit for hours and think of nothing or have an "empty mind." We have some tools such as a beginner meditation DVD or a brain-sensing headband to help you through this process when you are starting out. In general, the easiest way to begin meditating is by focusing on the breath — an example of one of the most common approaches to meditation: concentration.

CONCENTRATION MEDITATION

Concentration meditation involves focusing on a single point. This could entail following the breath, repeating a single word or mantra, staring at a candle flame, listening to a repetitive gong, or counting beads on a mala. Since focusing the mind is challenging, a beginner might meditate for only a few minutes and then work up to longer durations.

In this form of meditation, you simply refocus your awareness on the chosen object of attention each time you notice your mind wandering. Rather than pursuing random thoughts, you simply let them go. Through this process, your ability to concentrate improves.

MINDFULNESS MEDITATION

Mindfulness meditation encourages the practitioner to observe wandering thoughts as they drift through the mind. The intention is not to get involved with the thoughts or to judge them, but simply to be aware of each mental note as it arises.

Through mindfulness meditation, you can see how your thoughts and feelings tend to move in particular patterns. Over time, you can become more aware of the human tendency to quickly judge an experience as good or bad, pleasant or unpleasant. With practice, an inner balance develops.

In some schools of meditation, students practice a combination of concentration and mindfulness. Many disciplines call for stillness — to a greater or lesser degree, depending on the teacher.

OTHER MEDITATION TECHNIQUES

There are various other meditation techniques. For example, a daily meditation practice among Buddhist monks focuses directly on the cultivation of compassion. This involves envisioning negative events and recasting them in a positive light by transforming them through compassion. There are also moving meditation techniques, such as tai chi, qigong, and walking meditation.

BENEFITS OF MEDITATION

If relaxation is not the goal of meditation, it is often a result. In the 1970s, Herbert Benson, MD, a researcher at Harvard University Medical School, coined the term "relaxation response" after conducting research on people who practiced transcendental meditation. The relaxation response, in Benson's words, is "an opposite, involuntary response that causes a reduction in the activity of the sympathetic nervous system."

Since then, studies on the relaxation response have documented the following short-term benefits to the nervous system:

1-Lower blood pressure

2-Improved blood circulation

3-Lower heart rate

4-Less perspiration

5-Slower respiratory rate

6-Less anxiety

7-Lower blood cortisol levels

8-More feelings of well-being

9-Less stress

10-Deeper relaxation

Contemporary researchers are now exploring whether a consistent meditation practice yields long-term benefits, and noting positive effects on brain and immune function among meditators. Yet it's worth repeating that the purpose of meditation is not to achieve benefits. To put it as an Eastern philosopher may say, the goal of meditation is no goal. It's simply to be present.

In Buddhist philosophy, the ultimate benefit of meditation is liberation of the mind from attachment to things it cannot control, such as external circumstances or strong internal emotions. The liberated or "enlightened" practitioner no longer needlessly follows desires or clings to experiences, but instead maintains a calm mind and sense of inner harmony.

CHAPRER 2 : TECHNIQUES FOR BEGINNERS

This meditation exercise is an excellent introduction to meditation techniques.

Sit or lie comfortably. You may even want to invest in a meditation chair or cushion.

Close your eyes. We recommend using one of our Cooling Eye Masks or Restorative Eye Pillows if lying down.

Make no effort to control the breath; simply breathe naturally.

Focus your attention on the breath and on how the body moves with each inhalation and exhalation. Notice the movement of your body as you breathe. Observe your chest, shoulders, rib cage, and belly. Simply focus your attention on your breath without controlling its pace or intensity. If your mind wanders, return your focus back to your breath.

Maintain this meditation practice for two to three minutes to start, and then try it for longer periods.

CHAPTER 3: Meditation and sleep

It's no secret that meditation can help us sleep better. There are some specific meditative exercises that can help us nod off when our minds are in overdrive. In the exercise below, the meditation experts at Headspace share some insight for feeling more at ease when your head hits the pillow. Remember, this is not an exercise to make you go to sleep, but rather to increase your awareness and understanding of your mind at night. It just so happens that it often results in sleep.

Step 1

Once you're lying comfortably in bed, take five deep breaths, breathing in through the nose and out through the mouth. As you breathe in, try to get a sense of the lungs filling with air and the chest expanding. As you breathe out, imagine the thoughts and feelings of the day just disappearing into the distance, and any feelings of tension in the body just melting away. This will help to prepare both the body and the mind for the exercise ahead.

Step 2

Begin by checking-in -- how you're feeling --in both body and mind. Remember that in the same way you can't rush relaxation, you cannot rush sleep, so take your time with this part of the exercise. Don't worry if there are lots of thoughts whizzing around (this is absolutely normal). For now, just let them do their own thing. Whatever you do, avoid the temptation to resist the thoughts, no matter how unsettling or uncomfortable they may be.

Step 3

Next, become aware of the physical points of contact in a little bit more detail. Bring your attention back to the sensation of the body touching the bed, the weight of the body sinking down into the mattress. Notice where the points of contact are strongest -– is the weight distributed evenly? You can also notice any sounds or other sensations. Sounds can be especially disturbing when you're trying to go to sleep. At first it's helpful to recognize whether it's a sound you can change, or if it's something outside of your control, something you can do nothing about. Then, rather than resisting the sound, gently rest your attention on it, remaining present with the sound for 30 seconds or so, before bringing your attention back to the body.

Step 4

Now try to get a sense of how the body actually feels. At first, do this in a general way. For example, does the body feel heavy or light, restless or still? Then try to get a more accurate picture by mentally scanning down through the body, from head to toe, gently observing any tension or tightness. Invariably, the mind will be drawn to areas of tension, but you can relax in the knowledge that you are about to sleep and that the exercise will help to release those areas. You can do this scan several times, taking about 20 to 30 seconds each time. Remember to notice the areas that feel relaxed and comfortable, as well as any areas of discomfort.

Step 5

By now you will have probably already noticed the rising and falling sensation of the breath, but if you haven't, just bring your attention to that place in the body where you feel the movement most clearly. As always, don't try to change the rhythm of the breath in any way, instead allow the body to do its own thing. There is no right or wrong way to breathe within the context of this exercise, so don't worry if you feel it more in the chest than the stomach. Notice whether the breath is deep or shallow, long or short, smooth or irregular.

Step 6

As you watch the breath for a minute or two, it's quite normal for the mind to wander off. When you realize you've been distracted, that the mind has wandered off, in that moment you are back in the present, and all you need do is gently return the focus to the rising and falling sensation. You don't need to time this part of the exercise, you can just naturally move on to the next section when it feels as if a couple of minutes has passed.

Step 7

This next part of the exercise is about thinking back through the day in a focused and structured way. Begin by thinking back to the very first moment you can remember in the day, right after waking up in the morning. Do you remember how you felt upon waking? Now, as if your brain has been set to a very gentle "fast-forward," simply watch as your mind replays the events, meetings and conversations of the day. This doesn't need to be in detail, it's more of an overview, a series of snapshots passing through the mind.

Take about three minutes to go through the entire day, right up to the present moment. It might seem like a lot to fit into just a few minutes, but as I say, this is only an overview of the day, so don't take any longer than three or four minutes. After a couple of days you'll no doubt feel comfortable with the speed of it.

As the mind replays the day, there is the inevitable temptation to jump in and get caught up in the thinking. It's normal for the mind to wander like this at first, but obviously it's not helpful to get involved in new thinking at this time of night. So, as before, when you realize you've been distracted, gently return to the film playing back in your mind and pick up where you left off.

Step 8

Having brought yourself up to the present moment, you can now return your focus to the body. Place your attention on the small toe of the left foot and imagine that you're just switching it off for the night. You can even repeat the words

"switch off" or "and rest" in your mind as you focus on the toe. It's as if you're giving the muscles, joints, bones and everything else permission to switch off for the night, knowing they will not be needed again until the morning.

Step 9

Do the same with the next toe, and the next, and so on. Continue in this way through the ball of the foot, the arch, the heel, the ankle, the lower half of the leg and so on all the way up to the hip and pelvic area.

Before you repeat this exercise with the right leg, take a moment to notice the difference in the feeling between the leg that has been "switched off" and the one that hasn't. If there was any doubt in your mind about whether anything was actually happening as you do this exercise, you'll feel it now. Repeat the same exercise on the right leg, once again starting with the toes and working your way all the way up to the waist.

Step 10

Continue this exercise up through the torso, down through the arms, hands and fingers, and up through the throat, neck, face and head. Take a moment to enjoy the sensation of being free of tension, of not needing to do anything with the body, of having given up control. You can now allow the mind to wander as much as it wants, freely associating from one thought to the next, no matter where it wants to go, until you drift off to sleep.

It's quite possible that by the time you've reached this point in the exercise you will be fast asleep. If you are, enjoy the rest and sleep well. Don't worry if you're not asleep though -- it's not that you've done the exercise incorrectly. Remember that it's not an exercise to make you go to sleep, but rather an exercise to increase your awareness and understanding of your mind at night.

Want more tips on how to make meditation part of your day? Headspace is meditation made simple, accessible and relevant to your everyday life. Sign up for the free Take10 program to get the basics just right with guided audio programs and support to get your Headspace, anytime, anywhere on the Headspace app.

CHAPTER 4 : Better Sleep Through Meditation: 4 Techniques to Try Tonight

Moving to the desert may also help, but visualizing a peaceful scene is a good start.MasterfileAnyone who's ever experienced a fitful night of sleep knows that "just relax" is easier said than done. But do-it-yourself meditation practices may help you prepare for rest, and put worries or discomfort behind you.

These techniques work best when done right before bed, in a quiet, calming environment. But you can also practice them several times a day, recommends Joyce Walsleben, PhD, associate professor at New York University School of Medicine.

"If you can keep your stress levels under control during the day, you'll sleep better at night," Walsleben says. "You can even do them at your desk or on the train."

Abdominal breathing

Breathing from the abdomen and putting your attention on those breaths can help you relax both during the day and in bed at night.

Some people may enjoy lying in a dimly lit room, closing their eyes, or listening to soft music while focusing on their out breaths.

More techniques for better sleep

Yoga Moves for Better Sleep

While sitting or lying in bed, try placing your hands on your belly. "When you breathe in and breathe out, your hands may gently move," says Kathy Doner, MD, who has a full-time hypnotherapy practice in Sebastian, Fla. "Focusing on this movement gets your mind off of your busy thoughts and onto your body. You can distract yourself and bring yourself to a different place. It's very calming."

Some people imagine a calm scene to help them wind down at the end of the day. There are no rules about what you should imagine, so long as it's calming. Although clouds, the ocean, and mountains are common choices, you can focus on something as general or as specific as you want.

Mindful meditation

Focusing on different aspects of your life before bed can help you earn your rest, if you're able to let those thoughts goYou need to look at one thing at a time, which slows things down. Focus on an issue in your life, then let it go. The major learning experience here is letting go.

For some people, it may help to write in a journal during the day. For 15 minutes take those issues that run through your head at night and write them down,Then for the next 15 minutes make a plan and write that down too. At night when the lights are off, you can't do anything about it, but by processing things in the daytime, you can.

Counting down

While lying in bed, start by gazing upward. A little eye strain relaxes youTake an abdominal breath and hold it, and on the out breath, let everything relax. Repeat one or two times. You might then try imagining yourself walking down a flight of stairs or a gentle hill while counting down from 10 or 20, each number signifying your movement to a lower step, exhaling with each imaginary step.

You can also weave a number of these techniques together, You might start with your belly breath. then go to progressive relaxation, then down the stairs, then go to your peaceful place. You want to give people a lot of things to try.

CHAPRER 5: MEDITATION AND BRAIN

The meditation-and-the-brain research has been rolling in steadily for a number of years now, with new studies coming out just about every week to illustrate some new benefit of meditation. Or, rather, some ancient benefit that is just now being confirmed with fMRI or EEG. The practice appears to have an amazing variety of neurological benefits – from changes in grey matter volume to reduced activity in the "me" centers of the brain to enhanced connectivity between brain regions. Below are some of the most exciting studies to come out in the last few years and show that meditation really does produce measurable changes in our most important organ. Skeptics, of course, may ask what good are a few brain changes if the psychological effects aren't simultaneously being illustrated? Luckily, there's good evidence for those as well, with studies reporting that meditation helps relieve our subjective levels of anxiety and depression, and improve attention, concentration, and overall psychological well-being.

Meditation Helps Preserve the Aging Brain

a study from UCLA found that long-term meditators had better-preserved brains than non-meditators as they aged. Participants who'd been meditating for an average of 20 years had more grey matter volume throughout the brain — although older meditators still had some volume loss compared to younger meditators, it wasn't as pronounced as the non-meditators.

Meditation Reduces Activity in the Brain's "Me Center"

One of the most interesting studies in the last few years, carried out at Yale University, found that mindfulness meditation decreases activity in the default mode network (DMN), the brain network responsible for mind-wandering and self-referential thoughts – a.k.a., "monkey mind." The DMN is "on" or active when we're not thinking about anything in particular, when our minds are just wandering from thought to thought. Since mind-wandering is typically associated with being less happy, ruminating, and worrying about the past and future, it's the goal for many people to dial it down. Several studies have shown that meditation, through its quieting effect on the DMN, appears to do just this. And even when the mind does start to wander, because of the new connections that form, meditators are better at snapping back out of it.

5 Ways Policymakers Can Help Build A Future-Ready Workforce Today

A review study last year at Johns Hopkins looked at the relationship between mindfulness meditation and its ability to reduce symptoms of depression, anxiety, and pain. Researcher Madhav Goyal and his team found that the effect size of meditation was moderate, at 0.3. If this sounds low, keep in mind that the effect size for antidepressants is also 0.3, which makes the effect of meditation sound pretty good. Meditation is, after all an active form of brain training. "A lot of people have this idea that meditation means sitting down and doing nothing," says Goyal. "But that's not true. Meditation is an active training of the mind to increase awareness, and different meditation programs approach this in different ways." Meditation isn't a magic bullet for depression, as no treatment is, but it's one of the tools that may help manage symptoms.

Meditation May Lead to Volume Changes in Key Areas of the Brain

In 2011, Sara Lazar and her team at Harvard found that mindfulness meditation can actually change the structure of the brain: Eight weeks of Mindfulness-Based Stress Reduction (MBSR) was found to increase cortical thickness in the hippocampus, which governs learning and memory, and in certain areas of the brain that play roles in emotion regulation and self-referential processing. There were also decreases in brain cell volume in the amygdala, which is responsible for fear, anxiety, and stress – and these changes matched the participants' self-reports of their stress levels, indicating that meditation not only changes the brain, but it changes our subjective perception and feelings as well. In fact, a follow-up study by Lazar's team found that after meditation training, changes in brain areas linked to mood and arousal were also linked to improvements in how participants said they felt — i.e., their psychological well-being. So for anyone who says that activated blobs in the brain don't necessarily mean anything, our subjective experience – improved mood and well-being – does indeed seem to be shifted through meditation as well.

Just a Few Days of Training Improves Concentration and Attention

Having problems concentrating isn't just a kid thing – it affects millions of grown-ups as well, with an ADD diagnosis or not. Interestingly but not surprisingly, one of the central benefits of meditation is that it improves attention and concentration: One recent study found that just a couple of weeks of meditation training helped people's focus and memory during the verbal reasoning section of the GRE. In fact, the increase in score was equivalent to 16 percentile points, which is nothing to sneeze at. Since the strong focus of attention (on an object, idea, or activity) is one of the central aims of meditation, it's not so surprising that meditation should help people's cognitive skills on the job, too – but it's nice to have science confirm it. And everyone can use a little extra assistance on standardized tests.

Meditation Reduces Anxiety — and Social Anxiety

A lot of people start meditating for its benefits in stress reduction, and there's lots of good evidence to support this rationale. There's a whole newer sub-genre of meditation, mentioned earlier, called Mindfulness-Based Stress Reduction (MBSR), developed by Jon Kabat-Zinn at the University of Massachusetts' Center for Mindfulness (now available all over the country), that aims to reduce a person's stress level, physically and mentally. Studies have shown its benefits in reducing anxiety, even years after the initial 8-week course. Research has also shown that mindfulness meditation, in contrast to attending to the breath only, can reduce anxiety — and that these changes seem to be mediated through the brain regions associated with those self-referential ("me-centered") thoughts. Mindfulness meditation has also been shown to help people with social anxiety disorder: a Stanford University team found that MBSR brought about changes in brain regions involved in attention, as well as relief from symptoms of social anxiety.

Meditation Can Help with Addiction

A growing number of studies has shown that, given its effects on the self-control regions of the brain, meditation can be very effective in helping people recover from various types of addiction. One study, for example, pitted mindfulness training against the American Lung Association's freedom from smoking (FFS) program, and found that people who learned mindfulness were many times more likely to have quit smoking by the end of the training, and at 17 weeks follow-up, than those in the conventional treatment. This may be because meditation helps people "decouple" the state of craving from the act of smoking, so the one doesn't always have to lead to the other, but rather you fully experience and ride out the "wave" of craving, until it passes.

Other research has found that mindfulness training, mindfulness-based cognitive therapy (MBCT), and mindfulness-based relapse prevention (MBRP) can be helpful in treating other forms of addiction.

Short Meditation Breaks Can Help Kids in School

For developing brains, meditation has as much as or perhaps even more promise than it has for adults. There's been increasing interest from educators and researchers in bringing meditation and yoga to school kids, who are dealing with the usual stressors inside school, and oftentimes additional stress and trauma outside school. Some schools have starting implementing meditation into their daily schedules, and with good effect: One district in San Francisco started a twice daily meditation program in some of its high-risk schools – and saw suspensions decrease, and GPAs and attendance increase. Studies have confirmed the cognitive and emotional benefits of meditation for schoolchildren, but more work will probably need to be done before it gains more widespread acceptance.

Worth a Try?

Meditation is not a panacea, but there's certainly a lot of evidence that it may do some good for those who practice it regularly. Everyone from Anderson Cooper and congressman Tim Ryan to companies like Google and Apple and Target are integrating meditation into their schedules. And its benefits seem to be felt after a relatively short amount of practice. Some researchers have cautioned that meditation can lead to ill effects under certain circumstances (known as the "dark night" phenomenon), but for most people – especially if you have a good teacher – meditation is beneficial, rather than harmful. It's certainly worth a shot: If you have a few minutes in the morning or evening (or both), rather than turning on your phone or going online, see what happens if you try quieting down your mind, or at least paying attention to your thoughts and letting them go without reacting to them. If the research is right, just a few minutes of meditation may make a big difference.

CHAPTER 6: MEDITATION TO HELP YOUR MOOD

Meditation can alter your response to the major triggers of bad mood such as anxiety and stress. It has been proven to affect certain regions of the brain specifically linked with depression. But don't just take our word for it - these claims are backed up by credible scientific research, such as those conducted by the Harvard-affiliated Benson-Henry Institute for Mind Body Medicine.

Mood problems are more common than we think

Many of us believe that depression is only about those who are deeply discouraged. The most prevalent form of depression, however, usually leaves us able to continue our daily activities. The problem is we tend to go through our day often feeling emotionally numb. Sometimes we seem to disconnect from ordinary events and live on autopilot. Activities that used to be fun no longer are enjoyable. Socializing with friends can become dull or boring in many instances. Though much of our busy day can go well, when we are in a quiet part of our day, our unhappiness, anxiety, and feelings of hopelessness re-emerge.

How dark moods harms us?

Our mood can rob us of our satisfaction in living. Our ability to take pride in our work is diminished. Our relationships with key people are less satisfying. We often worry about our lack of skills and strengths. Feeling unworthy of success and happiness is common.

Chronic fatigue may accompany our day, and adequate sleep or naps do not seem to relieve it. Brain fog may occur, making it difficult to think clearly or exercise our creativity to cope with simple problems.

We may become more irritable and prone to bouts of anxiety or outrage. Thoughts of helplessness tend to recur, especially as we brood on our failures.

CHAPTER7: Meditation & Anxiety

Mindfulness meditation has long been known as an antidote for anxiety. However, the brain mechanisms involved in meditation-related anxiety relief were unknown. To isolate the brain mechanisms behind mindfulness training the researchers at Wake Forest Baptist employed pulsed arterial spin labeling MRI to compare the effects of distraction in the form of "Attending to the Breath" (ATB) before meditation training and to mindfulness meditation (after meditation training) on the state of anxiety in test subjects.

For the study, the researchers recruited fifteen healthy volunteers with normal levels of everyday anxiety. These individuals had no previous meditation experience or known anxiety disorders. All subjects participated in four 20-minute classes to learn a technique known as mindfulness meditation. In this form of meditation, people are taught to focus on breath and body sensations and to non-judgmentally evaluate distracting thoughts and emotions.

Anxiety was significantly reduced in every session that subjects meditated. Brain imaging found that meditation-related anxiety relief was associated with activation of the anterior cingulate cortex, ventromedial prefrontal cortex, and anterior insula. These areas of the brain are involved with executive function and the control of worrying. Meditation-related activation of these three regions was directly linked to anxiety relief.

There are many different types of meditation. In general, neuroscientists have been studying the benefits of both mindfulness meditation, in which you focus on sustaining attention and guiding thoughts; and loving-kindness meditation, in which you focus on compassionate thoughts towards yourself and others. Both types of meditation have been proven to change brain structure and have dramatic physical and psychological benefits.

For more tips and research on mindfulness and loving-kindness meditation please check out my Psychology Today blogs: Compassion Can Be Trained, Mindfulness Made Simple, Social Connectivity Drives the Engine of Well-Being and Mindfulness Training and the Compassionate Brain.

Mindfulness and loving-kindness meditation are secular. You don't need to become a Buddhist to incorporate mindfulness training into your daily routine. The Dalai

Lama has said that, "In the twenty-first century, even in countries with no previous tradition of Buddhism, interest is growing among ordinary people and scientists. The ethics and discipline described in the Vinaya are the foundation for training both in concentration (shamatha) and insight (vipassana)." He clarifies that with the help of focused concentration our minds have the ability to remain still and by applying analysis we can achieve higher understanding.

CHAPTER 8: Meditation Can Help Treat Depression

The ancient practice of meditation—
used for centuries in India and
China—now shows promise as a

treatment in the toolbox for depression.

The dozens of different types of meditation all seek a state of heightened awareness, says E. Robert Schwartz, MD, director of the Osher Center for Integrative Medicine at the University of Miami Miller School of Medicine, and that heightened awareness could have far-ranging benefits for people with depression and anxiety.

"There is a strong feeling in the neuroscience area and the psychology realm that meditation and meditative practices can change your brain physiology," Dr. Schwartz says.

Of course, you have to actually do it. "Learning how to manage your thoughts takes time, energy, and dedication," Dr. Schwartz says.

Keep in mind that adopting a meditation practice doesn't mean you abandon medications and other treatments for depression that you may already be using. "Meditation, particularly mindfulness meditation, has been shown to be helpful in treating depression, but it should be used as a part of conventional medical care under the supervision of a physician, and not as a substitute for conventional medical care," says Aditi Nerurkar, MD, medical director of the Cheng-Tsui Integrated Health Center at Beth Israel Deaconess Medical Center in Boston.

Here's a guide to some of the more popular and more studied types of meditation that can benefit people with depression.

Loving-kindness meditation

Loving-kindness meditation focuses on creating an attitude of love and kindness towards yourself and others. Several studies have found that people who practice this type of meditation have less depression, a more positive outlook, fewer negative emotions, and greater compassion.

Loving-kindness meditation may also help quell self-criticism, which underlies a number of different mental health disorders. One study found reductions in self-criticism lasted for at least three months after the actual meditation sessions had ended.

A related type of meditation, compassion meditation, stresses unconditional compassion and has also been linked with better mood and fewer negative feelings.

Mindfulness meditation

Mindfulness meditation might be considered the mother of all meditation. Many other types of meditation have stemmed from mindfulness, and it may have the most scientific evidence supporting it.

"Mindfulness meditation is a moment-to-moment awareness of the present moment," says Dr. Nerurkar. "It uses your breath to create an anchor to keep bringing your attention back to the present moment and help with cognitive retraining."

Studies have shown that mindfulness meditation may reduce depression, as well as anxiety and stress. The Society for Integrative Oncology recommends using mindfulness meditation to ease depression and anxiety in cancer patients, and studies have even documented ways in which mindfulness changes the brain.

Mindfulness-based cognitive therapy

This is a subset of mindfulness meditation that blends meditation with cognitive behavioral therapy or CBT. CBT is one of the most widely used forms of therapy for depression (and other mental health concerns) and focuses on changing damaging thinking and behavior patterns.

MBCT was first developed to prevent relapses in people with recurrent depression; more recent evidence suggests that it may also help people with active depression.

A recent study of the similar behavioral activation with mindfulness (BAM), which incorporates behavioral therapy with a mindfulness practice, found that it reduced symptoms of depression like changes in sleep, appetite, and mood. "BAM is an innovative type of intervention," says Samuel Y.S. Wong, MD, lead author of the study and professor and head of family medicine and primary health care at the JC School of Public Health and Primary Care at the Chinese

University of Hong Kong. "The two components are like 'yin' and 'yang.'"

Breath awareness meditation

Awareness of your breath is a fundamental component of many different forms of meditation, particularly mindfulness meditation.

"Mindfulness meditation uses the object of your breath to focus on, to help with mind training," says Dr. Nerurkar. Breath awareness meditation may also be called mindful breathing.

As little as 15 minutes a day of focusing on inhaling and exhaling can yield mood benefits, including lessened emotional reactivity. And you don't necessarily have to set aside special time to pay attention to your breathing: Many people find ways to incorporate awareness of their breath throughout the day. It can be done sitting, standing, or lying down, and with your eyes open or closed.

Yoga

Yoga combines physical postures with breathing techniques and meditation, and it seems to have an effect on depression and anxiety. Studies have found that Kundalini yoga in particular–which incorporates chanting–is helpful in the treatment of obsessive-compulsive disorder. Kundalini yoga includes specific techniques to manage fear, banish anger, and replace negative thoughts with positive ones.

Another study found that yoga, when combined with CBT, eased anxiety, depression, and panic while improving sleep and quality of life in people with generalized anxiety disorder.

Talk to your doctor before starting yoga. Unlike meditation, which is generally safe, yoga can cause injury, although this isn't common. Make sure you practice yoga with a qualified instructor.

Transcendental meditation

Transcendental meditation, or TM as it is known, has a large following around the world.

Instead of using the breath to anchor your attention, "transcendental meditation uses sound or a personal mantra, often one or two syllables, as the anchor," Dr. Nerurkar explains.

One study of teachers and staff at a residential school for students with severe behavioral problems–in other words, people with high-stress jobs–found that transcendental meditation improved stress, depression, and burnout, and that the benefits lasted four months.

Visualization

Many people find that focusing on pleasant images rather than negative ones stimulates calm. Visualization or guided imagery meditation can be led by another person, or you can direct your own session using one of scores of recordings available online.

Imagery can also be used to change how you recall negative memories. Imagining happy endings in place of such memories—a process called rescripting—resulted in better quality of life and self-esteem in at least one study. The participants were asked to revise past events in their imagination; visualize their moods as symbols or creatures, then transform them into something more positive; and find positive phrases and words to replace negative ones.

Body scan meditation

Body scan meditation involves focusing on different parts of your body sequentially. Like breathing awareness, you can do this lying down, sitting, or in other postures, and with your eyes open or closed. As you shift your attention to different parts of your body, you also focus on inhaling and exhaling deeply.

Body scanning seems to be linked with better observation of thoughts, feelings, and sensations and less intense reactions to stress.

One study that looked at body scan meditation among other forms of mindfulness found fewer depression relapses in people with bipolar disorder from a formal practice of just once a week.

Repetitive activity

Barack Obama once said he found washing dishes soothing. Cleaning up may not be a formal meditation practice, but repetitive activity—including scrubbing pots and pans—

may induce a certain calmer mental state, if you do it mindfully.

At least one study supports this idea, finding "mindful dishwashers" did show more mindfulness and less nervousness than those who didn't wash up mindfully.

"It's the repetitive action that doesn't require any real thought," says Dr. Schwartz. "It's the same as physical exercise. You're using the exercise or the manual labor as a way of calming your mind, focusing, and removing all of the extraneous thoughts that most of us have during waking hours."

Chanting

Many meditation traditions use chanting or periodic chimes of a gong as a way to focus the mind.

"Chanting is a modality to arrive at the same type of meditative state," says Dr. Schwartz. "You use that ... to gain your ability to focus."

One study found that "active-type meditative practices" like chanting and yoga seemed to activate parts of the brain involved in regulation of mood and emotional control.

To get more stories about mental health delivered to your inbox, sign up for the Healthy Living newsletter

Walking meditation

Walking, of course, is good for both your physical and mental health. But a walking meditation may take you to another level.

Aerobic walking coupled with Buddhist meditation three times a week for 12 weeks not only reduced depression but also improved flexibility and balance in a small group of older adults in one study. Meditating before or after walking (for as little as 10 minutes at a time) also lowered anxiety in younger adults in other research.

"Meditation is [about] learning how to not just focus your mind but also to relax your mind," says Dr. Schwartz. "You're learning now to bring [your mind] back to neutral," and you can do that not just while walking but with many forms of exercise, he adds.

CHAPTER 9: meditation and weight loss

Just as meditation can help us with stress, sleeping, focus, and much more, it can also have an impact on our relationship with eating and managing our weight.

When it comes to losing weight, we typically think of taking a spin class or opting for the salad instead of a burger for lunch. Consequently, it may seem counterintuitive to consider sitting in one place and focusing your thoughts, and doing a meditation for weight loss. These sorts of perceptions are only viewing part of the picture. Keep in mind that weight loss is not simply physical, and it's not simply black and white. As humans we're emotional beings, and acknowledging that fact is helpful in developing a healthy relationship with food, and potentially losing body fat or maintaining whatever weight is healthiest for our bodies.

Consider a 2017 meta-analysis of 19 different studies that found that typical weight loss methods (diet and exercise) work in the short term, but eventually the study participants' weight was gained back after the programs ended. On the other hand, weight loss protocols that included mindfulness interventions such as meditation (in addition to eating well and exercising), were seen to be more effective in reducing weight and keeping it off among study participants.

So, why is it possible that meditation helps when it comes to weight loss, exactly? There are physical and psychological factors at play. Another 2017 meta-analysis found that generalized meditation helped reduce cortisol and C-reactive protein levels. If our cortisol levels are consistently high, this is connected with the persistence of obesity over time, according to a 2017 study.

Psychologically, research shows that meditation may help squash overeating. A 2014 review compared 14 different studies and found that using mindful meditation as the #1 intervention decreased binge eating and emotional eating. Meditation has been shown to lower our stress levels. In fact, Headspace reduces stress in 10 days. This is important because stress is a contributing factor, causing many of us to overeat. Meditation teaches us to sit with and observe our emotions without passing judgment, instead of resorting to our go-to coping mechanisms like overindulging on food.

REF:

AMANDA GARDNER, ARTICLE IN HEALTH.COM

Alice G. Walton, ARTICLE IN FORBES MAGAZINE